Blood Type AB Meal Plan and Food List

A Custom Eating Plan and Blood Type AB Food, Beverage and Supplement Lists

Angela Casper

1

Table of Contents

Introduction

Eating is one of the most personal things we do each day. Food shapes our bodies, influences our minds, and even touches our spirits. And yet, for many, eating well feels more challenging than ever. We hear endless advice on diets, trends, and superfoods, but not all guidance fits everyone. Recently, there's been a renewed interest in how our blood type—the very blueprint of our biology—might affect our dietary needs and preferences. This book, "Blood Type AB Meal Plan and Food List," is here to help you explore a unique approach to wellness that aligns with the distinct characteristics of blood type AB.

Blood type AB is sometimes called the "modern blood type," as it's the newest and rarest blood group, found in less than 5% of the global population. Combining traits of both A and B blood types, those with AB blood often experience a blend of benefits and challenges, making it especially helpful to consider a tailored diet. Blood type AB individuals can show an adaptive immune system like type A but also carry some of the digestive strengths and weaknesses of type B. This dual nature influences the foods that work best for this blood type, which can be sensitive to certain foods but highly responsive to others.

In developing a meal plan specifically for blood type AB, it's essential to consider both scientific and practical aspects. While research on blood type diets is ongoing, many AB individuals report feeling healthier and more balanced when they eat in harmony with their blood type. This book doesn't promise to be a cure-all but instead offers a pathway to understanding how food choices might support overall well-being.

The "Blood Type AB Meal Plan and Food List" provides an organized, accessible approach to nourishing your body based on AB-specific guidelines. You'll find easy-to-understand explanations about why certain foods may benefit your blood type more than others and practical advice on meal planning to make this approach a lasting lifestyle. Each chapter will dive into what makes blood type AB unique, what to embrace, and what to limit in your diet. From immune-boosting fruits and vegetables to the best grains, proteins, and fats for your body, this book will guide you through crafting a balanced diet that works with—not against—your nature.

Eating according to blood type isn't just about restrictions; it's about optimizing what we eat to feel our best. Many people with blood type AB feel drawn to foods that are naturally rich in nutrients but gentle on the body. These foods nourish you without draining your energy. With this guide, you'll discover a variety of ingredients that align well with blood type AB and enjoy flexible meal ideas that can satisfy your taste preferences and nutritional needs.

Living healthily is not a one-size-fits-all journey. It's about respecting the individuality of your body and making choices that resonate with your unique biochemistry. In this spirit, "Blood Type AB Meal Plan and Food List" is written to help you make those choices confidently, blending scientific insights with practical, everyday guidance. Whether you're new to blood type diets or looking to deepen your understanding, this book is designed to be a trusted companion on your path to a more personalized approach to wellness.

Let's begin this journey together toward better health, vitality, and balance. As you turn each page, I hope you find inspiration, understanding, and a renewed connection to your body's innate wisdom.

Importance of Blood Type AB

Blood Type AB, the rarest of the blood types, holds a unique position in the landscape of human biology. It is often referred to as the "enigma" because it is the most recently evolved type, appearing less than 1,000 years ago. This blood type is fascinating not only because of its rarity but also due to the distinct characteristics and health implications it carries, blending the traits of both Blood Types A and B.

Genetic and Historical Significance

Blood Type AB is considered a biological enigma as it possesses both A and B antigens on the surface of its red blood cells. This mixed heritage offers insights into human migration and intermingling patterns. The presence of both antigens means that individuals with this type can receive blood from any other group in emergencies, positioning them as universal recipients, which is a significant advantage in medical scenarios.

Health Implications

The dual nature of Blood Type AB brings with it a complex set of health benefits and challenges. People with this type have a more tolerant immune system that can defend against several pathogens effectively. However, this same characteristic also makes them more susceptible to certain conditions like heart disease and cancer, which are less prevalent in people with other blood types. Their unique physiological makeup requires a balanced approach to diet and lifestyle, as recommended by the blood type diet advocates.

Psychological Traits

Individuals with Blood Type AB are often found to be adaptive, charismatic, and rational, yet they can also be unpredictable and tend to have complex emotional landscapes. They are known to thrive in situations that require diplomacy and are often considered excellent in roles that manage or mitigate conflict. This psychological profile can influence both personal and professional interactions, making them intriguing study subjects for psychologists.

Dietary Needs

The dietary recommendations for Type AB are as complex as their antibody makeup. They can benefit from a diet that includes a mix of vegetarian and moderate meat choices, which is unique among all blood types. Seafood, tofu, dairy, and green vegetables are highly beneficial for them, while red meat, kidney beans, and corn can be problematic. This balance is crucial for maintaining optimal health and preventing inflammation and other diet-related issues.

Exercise and Stress Management

For Type AB, stress management is crucial. They benefit significantly from calming exercises like yoga, tai chi, or meditation. These activities not only help maintain physical fitness but also contribute to emotional and mental well-being. Their natural inclination towards stress, influenced by their blood type, means that regular practice of these exercises can have profound health benefits, enhancing their quality of life.

The Importance in the Medical Field

In medical emergencies, the universal recipient capability of Blood Type AB can be life-saving, allowing transfusions from any other type without the typical risks of rejection. Additionally, understanding the medical tendencies of Type AB helps healthcare providers tailor preventive and therapeutic interventions more effectively, enhancing personalized medicine approaches.

Blood Type AB's rarity and complexity are what make it so fascinating. It serves as a reminder of our evolutionary past and the biological intricacies that continue to influence our health and behaviors in countless ways. For those who carry this blood type, embracing their unique biological and psychological traits can lead to a more personalized approach to health and well-being, aligning their lifestyle with their genetic predispositions to optimize their life experience.

Chapter 1: Blood Type AB Essentials

Characteristics and Health Profile

People with Blood Type AB have a fascinating profile, being the rarest of all the blood types. Known as the 'enigmatic' blood type, AB combines some of the traits of both Type A and Type B into a complex and often contradictory personality and physical profile. Understanding the essentials of this blood type can help those who have it manage their health more effectively and understand their unique traits.

From a health perspective, individuals with Type AB blood have a combination of the vulnerabilities associated with Types A and B. For instance, they may have the increased risk of heart disease seen in Type B, while also experiencing the higher rates of cancer that Type A is prone to. This requires a careful and balanced approach to health and diet to manage these risks effectively.

Type ABs are known for their empathetic nature, often being very emotionally sensitive and friendly. This makes them excellent at managing social situations and building networks but can also lead to stress as they navigate the complex emotions of themselves and others. Stress management is crucial for AB types. Techniques that emphasize relaxation and mindfulness, such as yoga or meditation, can be particularly beneficial.

Diet-wise, Blood Type ABs are somewhat of a paradox, being able to eat a wider variety of foods than other blood types, yet they need to manage the specific sensitivities inherited from their A and B ancestors. Foods that are beneficial for both A and B are generally good for AB, but they must be wary of meats and dairy products that can lead to sluggishness and higher cholesterol levels. A diet rich in seafood, tofu, dairy, and green vegetables is typically recommended, along with avoiding caffeine and alcohol, especially in stressful situations.

In terms of exercise, Type ABs benefit most from calming, centering exercises that maintain their emotional and physical balance. They thrive in regulated environments that ensure consistency and stability, which can be crucial in managing their stress levels and promoting overall well-being.

Overall, individuals with Blood Type AB have a complex health profile that benefits from a balanced approach to diet, exercise, and stress management, taking into account their unique genetic heritage and resulting health needs. By understanding and accommodating these needs, Type AB individuals can lead healthy, fulfilling lives.

Chapter 2: Food Guidelines

For individuals with Blood Type AB, navigating the dietary landscape involves a unique blend of challenges and opportunities. This blood type is rare and complex, merging the sensitivities of Types A and B. The ideal diet for Type AB is one that balances the tolerant digestive nature of Type B with the more sensitive gastrointestinal system of Type A.

Beneficial Foods for Blood Type AB

Dairy and Eggs: Type AB is the only blood type that can truly thrive on dairy products. Yogurt, kefir, and cultured dairy like cottage cheese are particularly beneficial due to their probiotic content, which can aid digestion and improve gut health. Eggs also serve as a versatile and beneficial protein source.

Seafood: Seafood is a superfood for Type AB, offering high-quality protein that's easy on the stomach. Salmon, sardines, cod, and mackerel are excellent choices, rich in omega-3 fatty acids that support heart health and cognitive functions.

Tofu and Other Soy Products: Soy proteins like tofu, tempeh, and edamame are excellent for Type AB. They provide essential amino acids without the fats associated with meat, making them ideal for maintaining lean body mass and supporting metabolic processes.

Vegetables: A wide variety of vegetables are beneficial for Type AB, with green vegetables leading the charge. Broccoli, kale, and spinach are not only easy to digest but also packed with vitamins, minerals, and antioxidants that can help combat the increased risk of diseases.

Fruits: While Type AB should be cautious with certain tropical fruits, more alkaline fruits like grapes, plums, and berries can be highly beneficial. These fruits are rich in antioxidants, vitamins, and fiber, promoting digestive health and preventing inflammation.

Grains: Unlike Type O, Type AB can handle grains more effectively. Oats and rice are particularly gentle on the stomach and can be excellent sources of sustained energy throughout the day.

Legumes: Some legumes are well-tolerated by Type AB, particularly lentils and beans, which offer a robust profile of fiber and protein, aiding in digestion and providing essential nutrients.

Incorporating Beneficial Foods

Creating meals around these beneficial foods can help those with Type AB optimize their health. A breakfast might include a serving of Greek yogurt with a handful of blueberries and a sprinkle of oats for a balanced start. Lunch could be a hearty salmon salad, rich in greens and dressed with olive oil and lemon. For dinner, stir-fried tofu with a mix of vegetables over brown rice can provide a satisfying and nutritious end to the day.

For individuals with Blood Type AB, embracing a diet that includes these beneficial foods can lead to improved health outcomes, better digestion, and an overall increase in vitality. It's about finding the right balance that caters to both the body's needs and the personal enjoyment of food, which is crucial for long-term adherence and wellness.

Navigating the dietary needs of Blood Type AB can sometimes feel like walking a tightrope, given its unique combination of traits from Blood Types A and B. While there are many foods that support the health and well-being of those with Type AB, there are also specific foods that are best avoided to maintain optimal health.

Foods to Avoid for Blood Type AB

Red Meat: While Type B can tolerate red meat, Type AB should tread carefully. The higher fat content and certain proteins in red meat can be difficult for Type AB to digest, often leading to sluggishness and fatigue. It's better to limit consumption and opt for leaner proteins.

Kidney Beans and Lima Beans: These beans contain lectins that can irritate the digestive tract of Type AB individuals, potentially leading to digestive disorders and an inability to absorb nutrients effectively.

Seeds and Corn: Certain seeds, like sunflower seeds, along with corn, can lead to digestive issues for Type AB. They may interfere with insulin efficiency and digestive stability, leading to fluctuations in blood sugar and digestive discomfort.

Wheat: While it's not necessary to completely eliminate wheat, Type AB individuals might find that large quantities of wheat can affect their calorie metabolism. This can lead to a slower metabolism, weight gain, and feelings of bloating or tiredness.

Caffeine and Alcohol: Type AB benefits from a calm and balanced nervous system, but caffeine and alcohol can disrupt this balance. Caffeine, particularly in coffee, can increase stomach acid and lead to gastrointestinal discomfort. Alcohol can also tax the digestive system and should be consumed in moderation.

Smoked or Cured Meats: These foods can contribute to stomach cancer in people with low stomach acid, which is more common in Type AB. Additionally, the preservatives and high salt content in these meats are not conducive to heart health.

Practical Tips for Avoiding These Foods

For those with Type AB blood, making informed choices at the grocery store and when dining out is key to avoiding these foods. Opt for whole, unprocessed foods as much as possible, and when in doubt, lean towards meals that are fresh and prepared with minimal additives.

Instead of reaching for a steak, a Type AB individual might enjoy a plate of grilled salmon or a hearty bowl of vegetable and tofu stir-fry. Snacking on almonds or carrots instead of corn chips or pretzels can make a positive difference in how they feel. When it comes to grains, alternatives like rice, quinoa, and spelt may be better tolerated and can replace wheat in many recipes.

By understanding and adapting to these dietary needs, individuals with Blood Type AB can significantly improve their digestive health and overall vitality. It's not just about avoiding what's harmful, but also about embracing a lifestyle that harmonizes with their genetic makeup, enhancing their health and enjoyment of life.

For individuals with Blood Type AB, finding a balance in their diet is crucial. This unique blood type combines the attributes of Types A and B, making it a versatile yet sensitive classification. While there are clear guidelines on what foods to embrace and avoid, there's also a category of foods that fall into a 'neutral' zone. These foods, neither highly beneficial nor particularly harmful, can be included in the diet of someone with Type AB without causing significant health impacts. Integrating these neutral foods allows for a varied and enjoyable diet while maintaining health and wellness.

Neutral Foods for Blood Type AB

Meats and Poultry: Chicken and turkey are considered neutral for Type AB. They don't offer the same benefits as seafood, but they also don't carry the risks associated with red meats. These can be a good source of protein when eaten in moderation.

Grains: While some grains like wheat might pose moderate issues, others such as rice, rye, and barley are neutral. They can be included in the diet without the adverse effects that might come from more problematic grains.

Legumes: Black beans, cannellini beans, and navy beans are neutral. They don't have the specific lectins that affect Type AB negatively, like kidney beans do, making them a safer choice for including in meals.

Nuts and Seeds: Unlike sunflower seeds, which should be avoided, nuts like almonds and seeds like pumpkin seeds are neutral. They provide a good source of fats and can be included in a balanced diet.

Fruits: Apples, bananas, and peaches do not offer the significant benefits that some other fruits might for Type AB, but they are also not detrimental. These fruits can be a part of a healthy eating plan, providing fiber, vitamins, and a natural source of sugar.

Vegetables: Potatoes and cabbages are examples of neutral vegetables. They don't provide the potent benefits of greens like kale or broccoli for Type AB, but they also don't cause harm and offer versatility and comfort in many recipes.

Dairy: Unlike other types where dairy might be a problematic area, for Type AB, most dairy products are neutral, including milk and cheese, which can be enjoyed without the adverse reactions other types might experience.

Incorporating Neutral Foods into the AB Diet

Including neutral foods in a diet can offer more variety, making it easier to adhere to dietary guidelines without feeling restricted. For instance, a lunch could include a turkey wrap with rye bread, a side of cannellini bean salad, and sliced apples for dessert. Such meals provide nutritional balance and dietary satisfaction without the highs and lows associated with more reactive foods.

For individuals with Blood Type AB, understanding and utilizing the list of neutral foods is crucial for crafting a diet that is both enjoyable and health-conscious. It allows for creativity in cooking and flexibility in meal planning, which are important for long-term dietary happiness and adherence. By skillfully incorporating these neutral items, people with Type AB can maintain a well-rounded diet that supports their unique physiological needs without feeling dietary fatigue or dissatisfaction.

Chapter 3: Nutritional Strategies

For individuals with Blood Type AB, a careful balance of nutrients and supplements can make a significant difference in their overall health and well-being. This blood type, a blend of A and B, benefits from a specific approach to nutrition that supports its unique traits and vulnerabilities. Understanding which nutrients are crucial and beneficial can help those with Type AB to feel their best, both mentally and physically.

Key Nutrients for Blood Type AB

Vitamin C: This essential nutrient is particularly important for Type AB because it helps combat the higher stress levels often associated with this blood type. Vitamin C supports immune function and is a powerful antioxidant that can help reduce inflammation—a common issue for Type AB. Foods rich in Vitamin C like oranges, red peppers, kale, and broccoli should be regulars in the diet.

Magnesium: Type AB individuals often deal with muscle relaxation and nerve function issues, making magnesium a vital nutrient. It assists in managing stress, improving sleep quality, and maintaining normal muscle and nerve functions. Foods like spinach, swiss chard, legumes, nuts, and seeds are excellent sources of magnesium.

Hawthorn: For those with Type AB blood, hawthorn can be a beneficial supplement. Known for its support of cardiovascular health, hawthorn helps regulate blood pressure and improves cardiac function. This is particularly valuable given the susceptibility to heart issues associated with this blood type.

Echinacea: Enhancing immune function is crucial for Type AB, and echinacea can be a helpful supplement. It boosts the body's natural defenses and is particularly useful during flu season or when surrounded by common colds, although it should be used judiciously as some individuals might develop allergies to this herb.

Valerian and Rhodiola: Stress management is key for Type AB, and these herbs can be beneficial. Valerian helps in promoting relaxation and sleep, making it ideal for dealing with the stress that Type ABs often experience. Rhodiola also aids in adapting to stress and enhancing energy and brain function.

Incorporating Supplements

While getting nutrients from food is ideal, supplements can also play a role in achieving the necessary levels of these nutrients, especially where dietary intake may not be sufficient. For instance, a Vitamin C supplement can be useful during times of illness or high stress when dietary sources are not enough. Similarly, magnesium supplements before bedtime can help improve sleep quality and reduce nighttime muscle cramps.

Practical Tips for Nutrient Intake

For those with Type AB blood, integrating these nutrients into daily life doesn't have to be a chore. Starting the day with a smoothie that includes spinach and citrus fruits can boost Vitamin C and magnesium intake. Snacking on almonds or pumpkin seeds can further increase magnesium levels throughout the day. Integrating a cup of hawthorn tea into the evening routine can support heart health and provide a relaxing end to the day.

Understanding these key nutrients and how to incorporate them into the diet can help individuals with Blood Type AB manage their unique health challenges effectively. Through a combination of a well-planned diet and strategic use of supplements, maintaining optimal health becomes a more attainable and straightforward goal.

Chapter 4: Weekly Meal Planning

Daily Meal Examples

Monday

- Breakfast: Greek yogurt topped with sliced almonds and honey, with a side of blueberries.

- Lunch: Turkey and avocado wrap with a whole grain tortilla, mixed greens, and mustard.

- Dinner: Baked salmon with a side of steamed broccoli and quinoa.

- Snack: Carrot sticks with hummus.

Tuesday

- Breakfast: Oatmeal with apple slices, cinnamon, and a splash of almond milk.

- Lunch: Lentil soup with a slice of spelt bread.

- Dinner: Stir-fried tofu with mixed vegetables (bell peppers, snap peas, carrots) over brown rice.

- Snack: A peach or some grapes.

Wednesday

- Breakfast: Smoothie made with soy milk, banana, spinach, and a tablespoon of flaxseed.
- Lunch: Salad with mixed greens, chickpeas, cucumber, and a balsamic vinaigrette.
- Dinner: Grilled chicken breast with sweet potato and green beans.
- Snack: A handful of pumpkin seeds.

Thursday

- Breakfast: Scrambled eggs with mushrooms and tomatoes on the side.
- Lunch: Quinoa and vegetable stuffed bell peppers.
- Dinner: Cod fillets poached in white wine with asparagus and wild rice.
- Snack: Sliced apple with a tablespoon of peanut butter.

Friday

- Breakfast: A smoothie bowl with kefir, mixed berries, and a sprinkle of chia seeds.
- Lunch: Spinach and feta stuffed chicken breast with a side salad.
- Dinner: Vegetarian chili served with a dollop of Greek yogurt and fresh cilantro.
- Snack: Cottage cheese with sliced pineapple.

Saturday

- Breakfast: French toast made with spelt bread, topped with fresh strawberries and a drizzle of maple syrup.
- Lunch: Sushi rolls featuring cucumber, avocado, and smoked salmon.
- Dinner: Beef stir-fry with a variety of vegetables and tamari sauce, served over soba noodles.
- Snack: A banana or a few squares of dark chocolate.

Sunday

- Breakfast: Pancakes made with rice flour, served with a compote of cherries and peaches.
- Lunch: Grilled shrimp over a kale and beetroot salad with walnuts and goat cheese.
- Dinner: Roast duck with braised red cabbage and mashed potatoes.
- Snack: A mix of dried apricots and almonds.

Tips for Successful Meal Planning

1. Variety is Key: Incorporate a range of beneficial foods throughout the week to keep meals interesting and nutritionally balanced.

2. Prepare in Advance: Use part of the weekend to prepare some meals ahead of time, like chopping vegetables or cooking grains and proteins, to make weeknight cooking easier.

3. Listen to Your Body: Adjust portion sizes and ingredients as needed based on how your body

reacts and what it needs. Some days you might need more energy or feel particularly drained.

By planning meals thoughtfully, those with Blood Type AB can enjoy a diet that supports their health without feeling restricted, leveraging the natural benefits of their compatible foods while minimizing adverse reactions. This approach not only sustains physical health but also enhances overall life quality by reducing stress around mealtime decisions.

Adapting to Various Lifestyles

Creating a meal plan that fits into the diverse lifestyles of individuals with Blood Type AB requires flexibility and an understanding that no two days are the same. Each person's daily routine, from the fast-paced executive to the stay-at-home parent, needs a tailored approach to nutrition that supports their activities and overall well-being. Here's how those with Blood Type AB can adapt their weekly meal planning to match various lifestyle demands:

For the Busy Professional

Busy professionals often struggle with finding time for balanced meals. For those with Blood Type AB, preparing in advance can be a lifesaver. Batch cooking on weekends and using slow cookers or pressure cookers can provide quick, nutritious meals without daily preparation. Portable breakfasts like yogurt parfaits or overnight oats are ideal for eating on the go. Lunches might consist of salads with multiple toppings and a protein like grilled chicken, which can be prepared in advance and packed for convenience.

For the Active Gym-goer

Individuals who have rigorous exercise routines need meals that support muscle recovery and energy replenishment. High-protein snacks, like a smoothie with whey protein and berries, are great post-workout. Incorporating lean meats, tofu, and legumes into main meals helps repair and build muscle. Hydrating foods like cucumbers and watermelon can help maintain hydration after intense workouts, along with plenty of fluids throughout the day.

For the Home-Based Worker

Those who work from home might find it easier to access a full kitchen, but the temptation to snack frequently can disrupt a structured meal plan. It's beneficial to structure meal times as if one were in an office setting to maintain regularity. Snacks should be health-focused, such as cut vegetables with hummus or a handful of nuts. Having clear meal and snack times can help avoid continuous grazing, which is common in home environments.

For the Parent Managing a Family

Parents managing both home and family needs can opt for versatile meals that please various palates while fitting the Blood Type AB diet. Dishes like stir-fries, pasta with plenty of vegetables, and homemade pizzas with different toppings can cater to different family member's tastes while being healthy. Involving children in meal preparation not only helps in teaching them about nutrition but also in making meal prep a family activity, reducing the burden on one person.

For the Retiree or Senior

For retirees or older adults, nutritional needs can include better management of chronic conditions and maintaining general health. Meals rich in fiber, moderate protein, and low in sodium are ideal. Cooking methods like steaming or broiling can enhance the natural flavors of foods without extra fats or salts. Soups and stews that can be made in batches and frozen in portions are convenient and can also be nutrient-rich.

General Tips for All Lifestyles

1. Flexibility: Be open to swapping meal components based on what's available seasonally and what fits into your day.

2. Preparation: Use tools like meal prep containers and planning apps to keep organized and on track.

3. Balance: Ensure each meal has a good balance of protein, carbohydrates, and fats, focusing on foods beneficial for Blood Type AB.

4. Mindfulness: Pay attention to how certain foods affect your body and mood. Adjust as necessary to optimize your health and energy levels.

Adapting meal planning to fit various lifestyles not only makes sticking to a dietary guideline easier but also more enjoyable. By considering individual needs and constraints, those with Blood Type AB can maintain a diet that's both satisfying and beneficial to their health.

Chapter 5: AB Diet Recipes

Recipes for Each Mealtime

Breakfast

1. Berry Yogurt Parfait: Layer Greek yogurt with blueberries, raspberries, and a sprinkle of granola.

2. Spinach and Feta Omelette: Whisk eggs and cook with fresh spinach and feta cheese.

3. Tofu Scramble: Sauté crumbled tofu with turmeric, onions, and spinach. Serve with whole grain toast.

4. Smoothie Bowl: Blend banana, soy milk, and a handful of spinach. Top with sliced almonds and chia seeds.

5. Oatmeal with Apples and Cinnamon: Cook oats with diced apples, sprinkle with cinnamon and a touch of honey.

6. Rice Porridge: Cooked rice simmered in almond milk with cardamom and topped with sliced peaches.

7. Turkey Bacon and Avocado Wrap: Wrap turkey bacon, avocado, and lettuce in a whole wheat tortilla.

8. Cottage Cheese with Pineapple: Bowl of cottage cheese topped with chopped pineapple and a sprinkle of coconut flakes.

9. Kefir with Mixed Berries: Pour kefir into a bowl, add strawberries, blueberries, and a drizzle of honey.

10. Pumpkin Pancakes: Make pancakes using rice flour and pumpkin puree. Serve with maple syrup.

11. Egg White Vegetable Muffins: Mix egg whites with diced peppers, spinach, and onions. Bake in muffin tins.

12. Soy Sausage and Egg Sandwich: Cook soy sausage, layer with scrambled eggs on a spelt bread bun.

13. Muesli and Soy Milk: Serve a bowl of muesli with soy milk, topped with sliced bananas.

14. Almond Butter Toast: Spread almond butter on toasted sprouted grain bread, top with sliced apples.

15. Breakfast Quinoa Bowl: Quinoa cooked with almond milk, mixed with dried apricots and pecans.

Lunch

1. Grilled Salmon Salad: Toss mixed greens with grilled salmon, avocado, cucumbers, and a lemon-dill dressing.

2. Turkey Lettuce Wraps: Fill large lettuce leaves with cooked ground turkey, shredded carrots, and cucumbers; serve with a tahini sauce.

3. Vegetable Stir-Fry with Tofu: Sauté tofu, broccoli, bell peppers, and snap peas in olive oil with garlic and serve over cooked quinoa.

4. Tuna and White Bean Salad: Mix canned tuna (in water) with white beans, sliced red onions, cherry tomatoes, and a vinaigrette.

5. Lentil Soup: Cook lentils with diced carrots, celery, and onions in a vegetable broth; season with thyme and black pepper.

6. Chicken and Rice Bowl: Top brown rice with grilled chicken breast, steamed spinach, and a sprinkle of sesame seeds.

7. Vegetarian Sushi Rolls: Roll sushi rice, avocado, cucumber, and cooked egg in nori sheets; serve with soy sauce.

8. Mozzarella and Tomato Salad: Layer slices of fresh mozzarella with tomatoes and basil leaves; drizzle with balsamic glaze.

9. Cottage Cheese with Chopped Vegetables: Mix cottage cheese with diced bell peppers, cucumbers, and tomatoes; season with a pinch of salt and pepper.

10. Egg Salad on Spelt Bread: Make egg salad with hard-boiled eggs, Greek yogurt, mustard, and chives; serve on toasted spelt bread.

11. Quinoa Tabbouleh: Mix cooked quinoa with chopped parsley, mint, tomato, cucumber, and a lemon juice dressing.

12. Pumpkin Soup: Blend cooked pumpkin with vegetable broth and onions, season with nutmeg and cinnamon; serve warm.

13. Grilled Shrimp over Kale Salad: Serve grilled shrimp over a salad of kale, beetroot, walnuts, and goat cheese with a light olive oil dressing.

14. Baked Cod with Olive Tapenade: Bake cod fillets with a topping of olive tapenade; serve with steamed green beans.

15. Stuffed Bell Peppers: Stuff bell peppers with a mixture of rice, ground turkey, tomatoes, and herbs; bake until tender.

Dinner

1. Sea Bass with Roasted Vegetables: Bake sea bass fillets and serve with roasted carrots, parsnips, and a drizzle of olive oil.

2. Beef and Broccoli Stir-Fry: Stir-fry lean beef strips with broccoli florets and a garlic soy sauce; serve over a bed of rice.

3. Turkey Chili: Cook ground turkey with tomatoes, kidney beans, onions, and a blend of chili spices; simmer until flavors meld.

4. Mushroom Risotto: Prepare creamy risotto using Arborio rice, a variety of mushrooms, vegetable broth, and Parmesan cheese.

5. Vegetable and Tofu Curry: Make a curry with tofu, spinach, and mixed vegetables; use coconut milk for a creamy texture.

6. Cod in Parchment: Bake cod fillets with sliced lemons, dill, and capers in parchment paper to seal in moisture and flavor.

7. Lamb Stew with Root Vegetables: Slow-cook lamb with turnips, carrots, and potatoes in a herbed broth.

8. Chicken Kebabs with Tzatziki: Grill chicken kebabs and serve with a side of homemade tzatziki sauce and pita bread.

9. Pumpkin Gnocchi: Serve homemade pumpkin gnocchi with a sage butter sauce and a sprinkle of grated nutmeg.

10. Ratatouille: Simmer zucchini, eggplant, bell peppers, and tomatoes with herbs for a classic French vegetable dish.

11. Baked Trout with Almond Crust: Oven-bake trout fillets with a crunchy almond crust, served with steamed asparagus.

12. Vegetable Paella: Cook a vegetarian paella with saffron rice, artichokes, bell peppers, peas, and olives.

13. Turkey Meatballs in Tomato Sauce: Serve turkey meatballs cooked in a rich tomato sauce over spaghetti squash.

14. Vegetable Lasagna: Layer roasted vegetables, ricotta, and mozzarella between sheets of pasta; bake until bubbly.

15. Grilled Halibut with Mango Salsa: Grill halibut steaks and top with a fresh mango salsa made with diced mango, red onion, cilantro, and lime juice.

1. Cucumber and Hummus: Slice cucumbers and serve with a side of hummus for dipping.

2. Greek Yogurt with Honey and Walnuts: Mix Greek yogurt with a drizzle of honey and a handful of walnuts.

3. Rice Cakes with Almond Butter: Spread almond butter on rice cakes and top with banana slices.

4. Turkey Jerky: Enjoy homemade or store-bought turkey jerky, a high-protein, low-fat snack.

5. Boiled Eggs: Have hard-boiled eggs on hand for a quick, protein-rich snack.

6. Fruit Salad: Combine favorable fruits like grapes, cherries, and apple for a refreshing treat.

7. Mozzarella Sticks: Enjoy fresh mozzarella sticks, either alone or with cherry tomatoes.

8. Pumpkin Seeds: Toasted pumpkin seeds make a crunchy, nutrient-dense snack.

9. Smoothie: Blend a smoothie with kefir, spinach, and frozen berries for a nutritious boost.

10. Edamame: Steam or boil edamame and sprinkle with a pinch of sea salt.

11. Cheese and Apple Slices: Pair slices of cheddar or mozzarella cheese with crisp apple slices.

12. Avocado Toast: Top whole grain toast with mashed avocado, a squeeze of lemon, and a sprinkle of salt.

13. Baked Kale Chips: Toss kale leaves with olive oil and salt, then bake until crisp.

14. Roasted Chickpeas: Roast chickpeas with olive oil and your choice of spices until crunchy.

15. Dark Chocolate Squares: Enjoy a few squares of dark chocolate as a sweet treat that's also rich in antioxidants.

Chapter 6: Lifestyle Tips

Dining out can sometimes feel like navigating a minefield, especially for those following a specific dietary plan like the Blood Type AB diet. However, with a bit of planning and savvy, eating at restaurants can be both a delightful and health-conscious experience. Here's how individuals with Blood Type AB can enjoy dining out without straying from their dietary needs.

Tips for Dining Out with Blood Type AB

Research Restaurants in Advance

Before choosing where to eat, do a little homework. Look up menus online and see if they offer AB-friendly options such as seafood, tofu, and a variety of vegetables. Many restaurants also cater to special dietary requests, so don't hesitate to call ahead and inquire about accommodating the Blood Type AB diet.

Choose Cuisine Wisely

Certain cuisines naturally align better with the Blood Type AB diet. Japanese, for example, offers numerous beneficial options like sushi (particularly those with salmon or tuna), sashimi, and edamame. Mediterranean cuisine is another great choice, with its emphasis on fresh vegetables, fish, and olive oil.

Communicate with Your Server

Once at the restaurant, be open with your server about your dietary preferences. Don't be shy about asking for dishes to be modified—such as requesting that a meal be prepared without certain ingredients like corn, kidney beans, or red meat, which are not ideal for Type AB.

Appetizers and Sides

Look for appetizers and side dishes that feature vegetables, tofu, or seafood. Salads are a good start, but always ask for dressing on the side to avoid any unwanted ingredients. Steamed or grilled vegetable sides are also a safe and healthy addition to your meal.

Be Mindful of Food Preparation

Type AB should avoid smoked or cured meats, so always opt for fresh or steamed options when available. Grilled items are typically a good choice, but make sure they aren't marinated in or covered with sauce that might contain ingredients that are best avoided.

Choose Beverages Carefully

Since caffeine and alcohol can adversely affect people with Type AB, opt for herbal teas, water with lemon, or even 100% fruit juices if available. If you wish to indulge in an alcoholic beverage, opt for those that are better tolerated like red wine, and always in moderation.

Handling Desserts

Desserts can be tricky. Opt for fruit-based desserts or even dark chocolate, which is beneficial for Type AB. Avoid desserts that are heavy in dairy and sugars, which might cause digestive stress.

Portion Control

Even when all the ingredients are right, overeating can still cause discomfort. Listen to your body and eat until you are satisfied, not stuffed. This is particularly important when dining out, where portion sizes can be larger than expected.

By keeping these tips in mind, dining out can be a pleasurable experience that complements the lifestyle of someone with Blood Type AB. It's about making informed choices that align with one's health needs without compromising on enjoying a meal out. With careful selection and a little creativity, maintaining a Blood Type AB diet while eating at restaurants is not only feasible but also enjoyable.

Combining Diet and Exercise

Type AB inherits some of the stress characteristics of Type A and the adaptability of Type B. This combination can lead to a unique set of stress-related health issues. Therefore, managing stress through a balanced diet and calming exercise routines is crucial.

Tailored Diet for Enhanced Performance

The Blood Type AB diet emphasizes a mix of plant-based and animal proteins, with a focus on seafood, tofu, dairy, and green vegetables. These foods not only cater to the digestive characteristics of Type AB but also provide the necessary nutrients for energy and recovery post-exercise. For instance, seafood and tofu deliver high-quality protein for muscle repair, while green vegetables offer minerals and vitamins to support overall vitality and immune function.

Recommended Exercise Regimen

Type AB benefits most from calming and centering exercises. Activities like yoga, Pilates, and Tai Chi are ideal as they help reduce stress and improve body strength and flexibility without overtaxing the system. These exercises promote a sense of balance and well-being, which is vital for Type AB's stress management.

While calming exercises are crucial, moderate cardiovascular activities should also be part of a

Type AB's routine. Exercises like cycling, brisk walking, or swimming for 30 minutes a day can help improve heart health and boost mood. It's important for Type AB individuals to monitor their body's response to exercise and adjust intensity to avoid exhaustion.

Strength Training Considerations

Strength training is beneficial for everyone, including Type AB, but it should be approached cautiously. Opt for lighter weights and higher repetitions rather than heavy lifting to avoid strain. Integrating strength training sessions a couple of times a week can help maintain muscle tone and bone density without causing undue stress.

Synchronization of Diet and Exercise

Planning meals around exercise sessions can optimize performance and recovery. Eating a light snack, like yogurt with berries, an hour before yoga or Pilates can provide a quick energy boost. After exercising, a meal rich in proteins and complex carbohydrates, such as a salmon salad with quinoa, can help repair muscles and replenish energy stores.

Listening to Your Body

Type AB individuals should be particularly attuned to their body's signals. If certain exercises lead to fatigue rather than energizing, it may be necessary to adjust the type or intensity of the workout. Similarly, dietary reactions should be monitored to ensure that food choices are supporting rather than detracting from overall health.

By carefully aligning their diet with a balanced exercise regimen, individuals with Blood Type AB can manage their unique health challenges effectively. This integrative approach not only enhances physical health but also promotes emotional well-being, creating a holistic sense of health that supports their complex nature.

Conclusion

As we reach the conclusion of our exploration into the Blood Type AB diet, it's clear that the interplay between genetics and lifestyle is more profound than we might have initially imagined. Understanding the unique characteristics of Blood Type AB has opened up a pathway to personalized health and wellness strategies that go beyond conventional nutritional advice.

The journey through the dietary needs, exercise recommendations, and the psychological and health profiles specific to Type AB highlights a tailored approach to well-being that considers more than just the nutrients on a plate. It embraces a holistic view of health that integrates mind, body, and spirit—a synergy that is particularly crucial for those with Blood Type AB.

For individuals with this rare blood type, the insights gained are not just academic; they are practical tools that can guide daily choices. The diet and lifestyle adaptations recommended for Type AB are not just about preventing illness but are also about enhancing life quality, managing stress, and optimizing physical health in ways that are uniquely suited to their biological makeup.

This personalized approach is a reminder of the beauty and complexity of human biology and how our individual differences require that we tailor our health strategies to fit our unique needs. It underscores the importance of ongoing research and dialogue about how we can better understand and support each blood type, particularly those as rare as AB, in finding their path to health.

As we move forward, let us carry the knowledge that while we may share many similarities with others, our individual health journeys are unique. The goal is not to strive for a one-size-fits-all solution but to craft a lifestyle that aligns with our intrinsic traits, allowing each of us to thrive. For those with Blood Type AB, and indeed for us all, understanding and embracing our individuality is the key to a healthier, more vibrant life.

Appendix

Proteins

- Seafood: Salmon, cod, mahi-mahi, red snapper, sardines, trout
- Poultry: Turkey, chicken (in moderation)
- Meat: Lamb, rabbit (consume sparingly)
- Dairy: Yogurt, kefir, mozzarella, ricotta, cottage cheese
- Tofu and other soy products: Tofu, tempeh, soy milk

Grains

- Safe Grains: Rice (brown, white, basmati), oats, rye, millet
- Flours: Rice flour, oat flour, spelt flour

Vegetables

- Highly Beneficial: Broccoli, beets, cauliflower, green leafy vegetables, garlic, onions, sweet potatoes

- Avoid: Artichokes, bell peppers, black olives, radishes

Fruits

- Beneficial Fruits: Grapes, cherries, pineapple, plums, cranberries, figs, grapefruit
- Neutral Fruits: Apples, bananas, pears
- Avoid: Mangoes, guava, bananas (if trying to lose weight)

Nuts and Seeds

- Beneficial: Peanuts, walnuts, almonds
- Avoid: Sunflower seeds, sesame seeds, poppy seeds

Legumes

- Good Options: Lentils, navy beans, soybeans
- Avoid: Kidney beans, lima beans

Oils and Fats

- Beneficial Oils: Olive oil, flaxseed oil
- Neutral Oils: Canola oil, cod liver oil

Spices and Condiments

- Beneficial: Ginger, curry, parsley, sage, garlic, horseradish
- Avoid: Vinegar, pepper (black, white, cayenne), capers, cinnamon

Beverages

- Recommended: Green tea, herbal teas (peppermint, raspberry leaf)
- Avoid: Alcohol, black tea, soda, caffeinated beverages